Massage Therapy and Cancer

By Debra Curties R.M.T.

Massage Therapy & Cancer
Debra Curties, R.M.T.
© Copyright 1999

To order copies, please contact:
Curties-Overzet Publications Inc.
1633 Mountain Road, Suite 12-179
Moncton, New Brunswick
Canada E1G 1A5
Toll Free Phone: 1-888-649-5411
Fax: 506-785-1908
Website: www.sutherland-chan.com/copi
E-mail: debra@sutherland-chan.com

ISBN 0-9685256-0-1

MASSAGE THERAPY AND CANCER

Introduction

The cancer diagnosis continues to be one of the most feared an individual can receive. Despite progress in research and medical treatment, the person with cancer experiences tremendous duress as a result of the physical and emotional impacts of having this disease. There are difficult decisions to make about the array of available treatments. As well, there are many personal ramifications of having cancer, some of which may substantially alter life as the person has known it. Treatment can be arduous and, without guaranteeing survival, may result in deformity or chronic disability.

The responsibilities of health care practitioners working with individuals who have cancer fall into three main categories: direct treatment, adjunctive therapy, and personal and lifestyle support. Massage therapists are not engaged in direct cancer treatment, but can play important roles in the other two categories of client care.

This booklet will present information about cancer, the most common cancer therapies, and the clinical issues for the massage therapist involved in the care of people who have cancer. The purpose is to establish a basic understanding of the disease and a set of guidelines from which the practising therapist can make informed and appropriate choices in massage treatment planning.

OUTLINE

Key Words

anaplasia
a tendency to regress to pre-differentiated or ancestor cell types; this reversion to earlier stage cells only occurs in cancerous growths

cachexia
a state of malnutrition, weight loss, and tissue wasting; frequently seen in advanced cancer; can occur as a result of both the disease and its medical therapies

chemotherapy
use of chemical or hormonal agents (antineoplastic agents) in an attempt to sterilize or kill disseminated cancer cells

malignant
in a general sense meaning harmful, growing worse, or having evil intent; is the term typically used to indicate that cancer is present

metastasis
refers to the movement of a disease process, especially of cancer cells, from one location in the body to another; metastasis to distant locations can occur via the bloodstream (hematogenous metastasis) or the lymphatic system (lymphogenous metastasis)

neoplasia
disorder of cell proliferation in which cells begin to reproduce outside the bounds of normal tissue controls and an abnormal tissue structure results

neoplasm/tumour
a mass of abnormal new tissue containing cells which are growing without compliance to the usual rules of tissue formation

oncologist
medical doctor who specializes in the treatment of cancer

palliative
in a general sense means used to relieve suffering; is often specifically used to connote care of the dying

parenchyma/stroma
the parenchyma is the group of functional cells which carries out the particular responsibilities of a structure; the stroma is the network of membranous connective tissue which gives the structure its shape and integrity

radiation therapy
the use of ionizing radiation as a localized therapy to sterilize or kill cancer cells

Learning Objectives

The purpose of this booklet is to provide the massage therapist with the tools with which to make appropriate clinical judgements when working with the client with cancer. Diagnosis and direct treatment of cancer are not within the massage therapy scope of practice; however the massage practitioner is frequently approached for massage therapy by individuals with this disease.

In the course of this reading the reader will develop:

1. an overview of the cellular behaviours, tissue changes, and general symptom picture associated with malignancies

2. an understanding of the rationales for the standard medical treatments for cancer, as well as their common effects and complications (short term and long term)

3. guidelines for the massage therapist considering working with a client who is also undergoing cancer treatment

4. guidelines for good case history taking

5. an awareness of the risk factors with respect to the possibility of massage promoting metastasis

6. general guidelines for massage therapy with cancer patients

7. specific guidelines for palliative care

8. an appreciation of what massage therapy can offer individuals with cancer

Three case studies, designed to help review your knowledge and apply clinical judgement, can be found at the end of the booklet.

WHAT IS CANCER?

Normal Cell Growth and Development

In the normal course of the cell life cycle, cells are produced and mature as needed, then die off as part of an aging or depletion phase or as the result of various types of injury. In most tissue types - with the exception of muscle and nerve which are formed of permanent cells - the dead cells are replaced by identical cells which occupy the same physical spaces and assume the same work responsibilities as their predecessors. This replacement process is known as **cell proliferation**, with the number and type of replacement cells being equivalent to those lost.

Cell differentiation is the process by which cells, within the limits of normal proliferation processes, transform into more evolved or specialized cell types. For each tissue type there are stem and progenitor cells (early stage cells) which give rise to the mature functioning units of that tissue. Even in adulthood a large number of ancestor cells are retained and can be signalled to generate a new crop of cells to maintain or replenish a tissue.

Within each tissue structure there is also a distinction between **parenchyma** and **stroma**. The parenchyma is the group of functional cells which carries out the particular responsibilities of the structure. The contractile fibers of a muscle and the secreting cells of a gland are both examples of parenchymal cells. The stroma is the network of membranous connective tissue which gives the structure its shape and integrity. These membranes act as the container and boundary for the functional cells. Contact with the stroma is essential for normal proliferation of parenchymal cells. This relationship ensures that tissue growth and repair processes give rise to the desired working structure.

Neoplasia

Neoplasia is a disorder of cell proliferation in which cells begin to reproduce outside the bounds of normal tissue controls. The resulting mass of new tissue, called a **tumour**, contains cells which are growing without compliance to the usual rules of tissue formation, and which continue to proliferate as renegades, even if the instigating stimulus stops.

It is typical of neoplasms that they manifest the following three disturbances of cell behaviour:[1]

- a disturbance in cell proliferation
- a disturbance in cell differentiation
- a disturbance in the relationship between parenchymal cells and their surrounding stroma

The result is a tumour cell population in which there is unregulated growth and disordered cell maturation. Often there is replication (reproduction) of one cell type in a number and manner which is completely inappropriate for the tissue structure.

Neoplasms can be either **benign** or **malignant.** This distinction is made on the basis of the characteristics and behaviour of the tumour cells. See the box below.

Distinguishing Features of Benign and Malignant Neoplasms

Benign	Malignant
• have an expansile growth pattern, enlarging locally within their host structures	• have an invasive growth pattern, overrunning host stroma and other tissue structures
• are usually contained within a capsule	• can invade body cavities and blood and lymph channels, leading to spread to secondary sites (**metastasis**)
• do not spread to distant sites	
• cells are usually fairly well differentiated	• cell replication is rapid and frequently abnormal
• cell turnover is slower	• poor differentiation and maturation of cells is typical, including a tendency to regress to pre-differentiated or ancestor cell types (**anaplasia**)

Signs and Symptoms of All Tumours

Benign and malignant growths are both parasitic on the nutritional and hormonal supplies of their host structures, impairing the health of nearby normal tissues. Both may also cause symptoms of abnormal tissue function because the tumour can promote increased or decreased output of tissue products. For example, in a gland responsible for saliva production, the presence of a tumour may cause the output of saliva to be either too little or too great, or to occur at inappropriate times. Also typical of both types of tumours is the potential to cause pain and altered function in the host tissue or neighbouring structures because of compression or obstruction. It is this last symptom category that often leads to diagnosis.

It should be noted that some members of the medical community use the term 'cancer' for any neoplasm, and distinguish the invasive type by calling it malignant cancer. However, the term cancer is most commonly used to signify malignant disease, and that is how it will be used in this text.

Characteristics of Malignancies

Malignant neoplasms are characterized by their invasiveness and ability to metastasize, and by the regressive (anaplastic) changes in their cells. They prosper because of their destructive and parasitic activities, their capacity to establish independent blood supply channels, their seeming ability to produce many of their own growth factors, and their lack of recognition of normal tissue controls. In illustration of the last point, non-malignant cells grown in culture dishes will stop reproducing when each cell is in contact with a neighbour. Malignant cells do not display this behaviour. Similarly, malignant cells do not require positioning on a basement membrane in order to proliferate.

Signs and Symptoms of Cancer

In addition to the signs and symptoms characteristic of all neoplasms, malignancies have many potentially far-reaching effects. In fact, the list is virtually unlimited, considering the numerous types of impact on host tissues and the possibility of diverse, often multiple, locations in the body. Some general trends in how cancer presents clinically are listed on the next pages. They are in categories which cover most of the types of signs and symptoms typical of cancers. Their implications for the massage therapist in practice will be elaborated later.

1. **Tendency to Cause Hemorrhage:** When a malignancy breaks through surfaces covered with epithelial cells (for example, the lining of the digestive tract), bleeding, which can be either slow or precipitous, often develops. Sudden hemorrhage is often the cause of early cancer death. Chronic blood loss may also induce severe iron-deficiency anemia. In addition, various ischemic occurrences can result (for example hemorrhagic stroke).

2. **Clotting Abnormalities:** In some cancers reduced clotting is seen, adding to the risk of hemorrhage. In others there is increased clotting activity, creating a concern about thrombosis and embolism.

3. **Immunosuppression and Infection:** Distinct from the roles chemotherapy and radiation usually play in suppressing the immune response, cancer itself has been shown to reduce all levels of immune system function. As a result of immunosuppression the person fighting cancer is susceptible to fungal and viral infections, tuberculosis, bronchopneumonia, and other such opportunistic infections. A tendency to promote allergic reactions or autoimmunity is expected in a percentage of cases, although the link to cancer has not been conclusively demonstrated.

4. **A Tendency to Enigmatic Tissue Damage and Poor Resolution of Injury and Illness:** Frequently what brings the individual to seek medical help is a puzzling injury (for example a spontaneous fracture), a persistent symptom, or failure to recover from a cold or other common illness.

5. **Fever:** Debilitating fever is frequently seen, with or without the presence of infection.

6. **Cachexia:** Cachexia is characterized by marked weight loss and tissue wasting. It is the result of loss of appetite (anorexia), malabsorption syndromes which occur with some cancers and cancer therapies, and high volume consumption of nutrients by the tumour(s). Some research is also being directed at determining whether tumours may release toxins which are detrimental to general tissue health.

7. **Nausea, Vomiting, Diarrhea:** In addition to the fact that medical treatment modalities can produce this type of symptom, cancer-caused digestive disturbances are common, especially, but not exclusively, with gastrointestinal tract malignancies.

8. **Abnormal Hormone Secretion:** Tumours may give rise to abnormal levels of hormone production. For example, the presence of a tumour in an adrenal gland may result in elevated adrenalin levels. Malignant tumours may also produce peptides and hormonal products which are not typical of the original tissue. This occurs as a result of cellular abnormalities characteristic of cancer and is called **ectopic hormone production**. It is clinically significant because of the possibility of unusual physical or psychoemotional symptoms.

9. **Pain:** Pain is not typical in the majority of early stage cancers. As the cancer progresses, approximately 40% of individuals in the intermediate stages and 60-80% of those in the advanced stages will have pain severe enough to adversely impact their physical and psychological wellbeing.[2] Cancer pain is often described as being subjectively more intense because of the psychological stresses associated with the disease.

10. **Skin Lesions:** Various skin lesions may occur with the presence of cancer in the body. The most common include pigmentation changes, red flushing (erythema), and increased susceptibility to skin infections. Dermatomyositis, ordinarily not a common condition, is associated with a surprisingly high number of malignancies. Many authors offer statistics on this, suggesting from 15% to 50% incidence in all individuals with cancer. Dermatomyositis presents as proximal pain and weakness, especially of the shoulder and hip girdles, in association with a red/purple rash over the face, chest, posterior neck, and extensor surfaces of the limbs.

11. **Nervous System Complications:** 1 person in 5 with disseminated cancer develops major signs of nervous system dysfunction, either via brain metastasis (most common), side effects of medical treatment, or metabolic effects of the disease on nervous system function[3] (for example, electrolyte imbalances causing impairment of neuron transmission). The range of possible CNS symptoms is vast. The most common early signs of brain metastasis are: changes in alertness, intellectual impairment, and gait abnormalities; of meningeal metastasis: confusion, irritability, headaches, and vomiting; of spinal cord metastasis: back pain, weakness, and muscle atrophy. Altered sensation may be noticed in any of the above. In all cases the symptoms may emerge slowly or quite rapidly. Sudden brain metastasis may mimic stroke. Cranial neuropathies (for example trigeminal neuralgia) are also common; however brain infections are not typical.

12. **Vital Organ Complications:** The four other vital organs (in addition to the brain) are the liver, heart, kidneys, and lungs. All are susceptible to metastasis. They are also frequently subjected to considerable duress from the exigencies of the disease and standard medical treatments. The possibility of diminished or abnormal function in these organ systems must always be considered.

Cancer Therapies

The large majority of individuals with cancer will have a history of or current involvement with one or more types of cancer treatment. The purpose of this section is to provide a foundation for understanding the common medical treatment approaches. Beyond helping the therapist to empathize to some extent with the experience of the client, such understanding is important for massage treatment planning.

This text does not attempt to address the group of medical and non-medical treatments presently referred to as alternative therapies. In the medical context the term 'alternative' implies a type of direct treatment which may be used in the place of more common methods. Examples include: hyperthermia (raising the temperature of the tumour), electrical current tumour stimulation, and a variety of experimental diets, drugs, and substances. The choice not to address these treatment options here does not reflect on their merits. It is difficult to make conclusive statements about the place of most such therapies in the cancer treatment picture at this time. The massage practitioner who encounters less orthodox treatment choices in the case presentation of a client must seek out sufficient information/opinion to be able to design a compatible treatment plan.

Many adjunctive therapies are now being incorporated into cancer treatment plans, and with increasing acceptance. Examples include: nutritional therapy, relaxation, visualization, massage therapy, acupuncture, and psychotherapy. The term 'adjunctive' in this context implies use along side of other, usually more conventional, treatment approaches.

Incorporation of adjunctive therapies in a treatment protocol may be justified by medical personnel because they enhance the person's physical resilience and tolerance of treatment. From the perspective of the practitioners of these therapies and the individuals who seek them out, several other benefits have also been suggested. The role of adjunctive therapies, particularly massage therapy, will be considered shortly.

Surgery

The primary goal of cancer surgery is to remove localized cancers. If a tumour has been found early enough, surgery may result in a cure. The surgical procedure usually involves removal of the cancerous tissue, some adjacent normal tissue, and frequently regional lymph nodes. Sometimes 'debulking' operations are undertaken, in which large tumours are excised in the hope that reducing the tumour load will make it possible for the body's defences and the cancer therapies to handle the remaining smaller growths.

Despite some controversy about the extensiveness required in cancer operations (for example radical mastectomy versus lumpectomy), surgery is still considered the most effective of the current medical procedures.[4] Surgery preceded or followed by radiation and/or chemotherapy remains the most consistently used treatment approach.

Surgery may also be performed for palliative reasons, in other words for relief of suffering. Such surgical interventions are not intended as primary cancer therapy. Examples include: removal of obstructions (for example in the bowel), pain control procedures, and removal of cancerous tissues which induce complications like hemorrhage or hormone abnormalities. The benefits versus risks of these operations are not easily generalized and their utility is determined on a case-by-case basis.

Radiation Therapy

The aim of radiation therapy is to render cancer cells sterile, or incapable of reproduction. Radiation exposure can cause immediate cell death if the dose is high enough, but it is not safe or necessary to attempt to kill all cancer cells present as long as enough damage can be inflicted to stop proliferation.

Most radiation treatment protocols are organized in regularly spaced sessions (for example 5 days on, weekend rest period, 5 more days, and so on) to attain a cumulative dosage deemed most destructive to the cancer. Radiation is considered best suited to small tumour situations and is frequently used to 'clean up' after surgery, or before surgery to shrink a tumour to a more operable size.

It is still not certain exactly how radiotherapy affects the cell. It either disrupts existing DNA, RNA, or proteins in the cell, all of which are essential for cell replication, or it interferes with synthesis of these products.

Several drugs have been found to enhance cellular radiosensitivity and may be used as part of the treatment protocol.

At a certain dose threshold, all cells sustain some degree of radiation injury. Particularly vulnerable are cells in the process of reproducing. In addition, each type of cell has its own sensitivity level for sterilization, so dosages must be determined by the cancer type.

The difficulty is that all cells in the irradiated zone will be affected by the treatment - especially if they are replicating - since the cancerous cells cannot be separately targeted. The argument for the usefulness of radiation is based on the following rationales:

- The ratio of cells which are reproducing at any given point is generally much higher in cancerous growths than in normal tissues, making them more vulnerable to the radiation.

- Normal tissues, which are organized into functional structures, are believed to be better able to cope with cell loss, and more capable of replacing missing cells in a purposeful way. Cancer masses do not reconstruct themselves as a unit following cell loss; they simply keep proliferating as they are able.

Limitation on radiation doses is ultimately determined by the tolerance of the normal tissues. It would not be meaningful to eliminate the cancer if life cannot be sustained or if remaining vital tissues are damaged beyond a reasonable capacity to return to function.

Radiation therapy is controlled as carefully as possible to restrict normal tissue exposure. Radiation sites are ink-marked or tattooed for future reference, and these marks must not be tampered with for the duration of the treatment plan.

The most common effects of radiation on normal tissues are: skin lesions, which are in essence burns with associated pain and inflammation followed by epidermal desquamation and itching; localized hair loss; bone marrow suppression; enteritis, possibly with vomiting or diarrhea; mucous membrane irritation or suppression (for example, sinus congestion or dryness if the face is irradiated); and the possibility of glandular dysfunction. Generalized fatigue, a result of the overall drain on the body's resources, is usually reported by individuals undergoing radiation treatment. These occurrences are all expected to resolve in time after the treatment ceases.

Some more long-term, or perhaps permanent, tissue changes can be seen following radiation therapy. The affected skin surface may remain hypersensitive to temperature and pressure for some time. There may be permanent weakening of local bones and soft tissue structures (for example tendons, joint cartilage). Radiation of the vital organs, whether direct or indirect - lung and heart tissue may be exposed to radiation during breast cancer treatment, for example - can result in reduced function. Some risk of later development of radiation induced cancer in the treated normal tissues is always present. Also, radiation of the ovaries or testes frequently results in infertility.

Chemotherapy

The goals of chemotherapy are similar to those of radiation therapy. Chemotherapy is the use of chemical agents (antineoplastics) to kill or sterilize cancerous cells. Many of these agents are toxic substances which promote desired types of cell damage. Hormonal manipulation of tumour cells is also used.

Chemotherapy is employed in similar circumstances and often in conjunction with radiation. Because the antineoplastic substance enters the general circulation, chemotherapy is most likely to be incorporated into the treatment protocol if the cancer is disseminated, or if the risk of existing metastasis seems high. Although most often given intravenously, the agents may be administered orally, intra-arterially, or intramuscularly, usually in a schedule designed to create a cumulative sub-lethal dose which is as high as possible.

There are some instances in which chemotherapy is used to treat a tumour locally. Substances may be injected directly into the tumour. A technique called **perfusion re-circulation** may also be employed. In this procedure the individual's blood is re-circulated through the tumour vicinity by means of a circulatory loop created through an equipment linkage between local arterial and venous channels. The chemotherapeutic substance is injected into the loop. Although some entry of the agent into the general circulation will occur, a highly concentrated dose can be directed at the tumour. This type of regional treatment is not as common as the generalized applications, however, where all body tissues are exposed as the agent circulates.

Certain cell types are more sensitive to specific cytotoxic (cell damaging) agents, and the antineoplastics used are determined as much as possible by the cancer type. Refinements in chemotherapy are leading to improved 'targeting' of tumours in some cancers, where the abnormal cells are actually being attacked on the basis of their particular chemical properties or hormonal vulnerabilities. In most cases, however, it remains true that all cells in the body are subject to damage. Treatment rationales are essentially the same as for radiation therapy. Dosages are carefully controlled to provide maximum sterilization of cancerous cells within the limits of what can be tolerated by the normal tissues.

Individuals receiving chemotherapy treatment usually experience side effects of varying severity. Typical side effects include: nausea, vomiting, and diarrhea; hair loss; inflammation and bleeding in structures lined by rapidly reproducing epithelial cells such as the respiratory and digestive tracts; pronounced fatigue and malaise; pain; immunosuppression; and bone marrow suppression, with the possibility of sufficient loss of red blood cell production to induce severe anemia. Fear of the secondary effects of chemotherapy may be a significant factor in itself, inducing a high level of anxiety and perhaps exacerbating symptoms.

Long term effects of chemotherapy frequently include infertility, induced menopause, arthritic changes in joints, and a degree of vital organ damage that may or may not be clinically significant.

Effects of Radiation and Chemotherapy

It is often noted that the effects of radiation and chemotherapy, particularly in combination, are very similar to the signs and symptoms of cancer. For this reason it would be useful to consult the **General Symptom Trends in Cancer** list on pages 10 and 11. This tendency to produce similar signs and symptoms can lead to difficulties in establishing causal relationships for clinical occurrences seen in the person with cancer. From the point of view of the massage therapist considering treatment plan designs, some effects are of particular note. These include:

- tissue fragility, especially of epithelial structures like skin

- a tendency to hemorrhage, perhaps with reduced clotting ability

- risk of thromboembolism

- increased risk of infection

- slower healing times

- fatigue and malaise, with the possibility that standard massage treatment approaches may be overtaxing

- electrolyte imbalances which can result in cardiac dysrhythmias or altered neuron firing (possibly producing alterations in alertness or mood, sensation, reflex responses, muscle power, coordination, pain levels)

- the possibility of weakness or overstress of one or more of the vital organs

- pain

CLINICAL CONSIDERATIONS FOR THE MASSAGE THERAPIST

We will now begin to look at how this information about cancer and the common cancer treatments impacts on massage therapy. It is not required that the massage practitioner be an expert on the numerous types of cancer or on direct treatment modalities. It is reasonable to expect, however, that a massage therapist treating individuals with cancer will be sufficiently knowledgeable to be able to pursue the necessary information about each client's case and to make safe and appropriate treatment decisions. There are several questions which must be considered as part of the judgement process.

Could Massage Therapy Promote Cancer Metastasis?

Cancers spread from the original tumour site by four mechanisms:

- progressive direct local invasion of nearby structures
- through body cavities
- to distant sites via the bloodstream (*hematogenous metastasis*)
- to distant sites via the lymphatic system (*lymphogenous metastasis*)

The processes involved in metastasis are highly complex and still incompletely understood despite a great deal of research. This ongoing research is motivated by the fact that metastasis is almost always what causes cancer death. "Modern surgery and/or radiation therapy successfully eradicates the majority of primary tumours but the inability to control metastases is the principal reason why there has been little progress in reducing cancer mortality in the last 30 years."[5] This statement, written a decade ago, still holds an unfortunate degree of truth and explains why prognosis is typically based on degree of, or likelihood of, metastasis in a case.

The majority of lethal cancers involve blood circulation metastasis. Currently, there is a good prognosis with prompt treatment in cancers limited to local lymph node spread, but with increasingly distant lymphogenous metastasis the survival rate decreases, especially as the neoplastic cells eventually join the bloodstream.

Massage therapy and associated modalities like hydrotherapy and remedial exercise can act as strong stimuli to blood and lymph flow, so it is important to take a serious look at whether massage therapy could promote metastatic processes.

Events in Distant Metastasis[6,7]

Hematogenous Spread	Lymphogenous Spread
1. Cell shedding from the primary tumour.	1. Cell shedding from the primary tumour.
2. Poor quality of tumour blood vessels facilitates permeation; cells pass through the blood vessel walls into the lumina, and hence the blood.	2. Movement of cells into the interstitial space of the host or nearby structures.
3. Transport of tumour cells in the bloodstream. Cells may aggregate, increasing their chance of success.	3. Cells penetrate into lymph capillaries, or are picked up by them, and enter the small lymph vessels.
4. Impact in a capillary network, usually the first encountered.	4. Travel to regional lymph nodes.
5. Destruction, or adherence to blood vessel walls, or continued travel to subsequent sites.	5. Destruction by immune system cells or proliferation in the node. Note that cells can enter the bloodstream via the nodal capillaries.
6. Penetration through capillary walls to tissue interstitium.	6. Passage to right lymphatic and thoracic ducts.
7. Secondary tumour growth.	7. Entry to bloodstream. See Hematogenous Spread.

The set of events and possibilities in distant metastasis is complex. At each stage the body's defence systems are capable of eradicating the malignant cells. Evidence suggests that far more are killed than survive. The 'successful' cells overcome a harrowing set of challenges. In one study (Fidler, 1978)[8] where injected radiolabeled cancer cells were monitored, most cells were destroyed within 24 hours, and after 3 days less than 0.1% remained viable. This result has been substantiated in several high quality studies.[9]

We can only surmise the role massage therapy could play in these events, since research on the subject has not been conducted. Clinically based consultation with physicians and careful examination of known data permits some presumably reasonable conclusions to be drawn. However, it must be noted that the current lack of certain knowledge may pose some degree of risk to our clients.

We will consider the metastasis process to be occurring in three principal stages and examine the potential impact of massage therapy at each stage.

Stage 1.
Cell Shedding from the Primary Tumour

Tumour cells for the various cancer types have their own characteristic rates and time frames for metastatic development. It is possible that only a certain percentage of cells are capable of the 'splitting off' mechanism, and that this percentage varies in different cancers. These factors are beyond the control of the massage therapist.

The question remains, however: Could direct pressure or another strong stimulus, such as intense hydrotherapy, enhance the potential for cell shedding from a malignant tumour? One instructive reference was found in the physiotherapy context. "This process [of cancerous cells entering the bloodstream] is influenced by several factors, such as biomechanical processes or gross mechanical manipulation, which can drive a large number of cells into circulation."[10] The implication is that sufficient direct pressure will traumatize the tumour and promote release of cells. It may also be inferred by "biomechanical processes" that an intense movement modality (for example, passive forced stretching) or a highly stimulating local hydrotherapy application might be unsafe.

In response to a question from a physician, this medical opinion was offered in the Journal of the American Medical Association in 1977: "I firmly believe that heat and massage should not be used if there is any possibility that a primary or metastatic neoplasm exists in the skin or subcutaneous tissue at the site of application."[11] This is an old source, but it reflects a current concern. The implication is that the closer the cancer is to the skin surface, the greater the risk from massage therapy.

It would be more satisfying to be able to consider a larger volume of research and opinion. However, the possibility clearly exists that some components of massage treatment, if applied locally and with sufficient intensity, especially to a superficial tumour, could provoke cell shedding.

Stage 2.
Circulation in the Blood or Lymph Channels

As previously discussed, it has been accepted that the rate of survival of metastatic cells in the bloodstream is somewhere under one per cent. This extremely high mortality rate is hypothesized to be the result of several hostile factors. These include attack by the host's immune system, incapacity of the sessile (not designed for movement) cancer cells to absorb nutrients while in circulation, and trauma from continuous movement.

The relevant question for massage therapy could be stated as: Could an increase in blood or lymph flow aid the survival of circulating cancerous cells? No specific reference was found in answer to this question, but several pieces of related research and opinion would suggest not. The massive destruction of cancer cells in the blood and lymph indicates that these environments are always highly antagonistic. Given these hostile factors, increased speed or volume of flow would be as likely to jeopardize cell survival as support it.

If an increased risk does exist, massage would not be isolated in creating this type of effect. Were it to be true that stimulation of the circulation encourages metastasis, hot showers, exercise, sexual activity, and many other aspects of daily life would confer equivalent risks. Individuals with cancer are almost always encouraged to exercise and remain as active they can; such advice from the medical community would seem to place other values ahead of a risk of promoting metastasis from a general circulation increase. About the role of exercise specifically, Dr. Carl Simonton makes the following statement: "The overall picture is that people engaged in regular exercise programs tend to develop a healthier psychological profile in general - one often identified with a favourable prognosis for the course of the malignancy."[12] Similar claims can likely be made about regular massage therapy. One study[13] makes reference to the following effects of repeated massage treatments for cancer clients: promotion of the relaxation response, decreased muscle tension, nausea, anxiety, and psychological distress, and reduction in feelings of isolation.

It has also been argued that promoting better circulatory efficiency, especially in lymph flow, may aid the host immune response and therefore encourage better eradication of cancerous cells. These arguments are presently based on personal opinion and clinical observation. Current research on manual lymph drainage techniques may offer some answers.

Stage 3.
Implantation at a Secondary Site

Here we are addressing the potential for implantation of surviving metastatic cells once they reach the capillary network of a possible secondary site. Although there is also high cancer cell morbidity at this stage because of host immune cell activity, could the likelihood of their enduring and proliferating in the tissue somehow be increased by massage therapy? The possibility that such a risk exists has not been proven or disproven by research. The concern hinges on the fear that massage therapy techniques could mechanically cause more cells to lodge in capillary beds and hence increase the possibility of successful implantation.

Pushing blood in greater volume or at higher pressure toward capillary beds can result in greater arrest of tumour cells. However, it has been repeatedly shown that despite the fact that cancer cells will impact in the first small vessels encountered (as with other emboli), they do not necessarily develop at those sites[14,15]. While there is the possibility of randomized distribution of metastases in a small percentage of cancers, the pattern of metastasis is usually seen to be characteristic for each cancer and is based more on tissue affinities. Some of the reasons for this are believed to be:[16]

- the 'homing' ability of some cancers – they prefer certain tissue environments
- some cancers do not have the enzymes needed to destroy some tissue matrices and/or basement membranes
- some cancers have an affinity for endothelium
- some organs do not have the right growth factors for some cancers

In other words, the end result does not reflect secondary tumor growth in nearest capillary beds, but rather a preference to become established in specific tissues for other reasons.

Patterns of metastasis formation are well documented for most cancers, and therefore are easily researched by the massage therapist. A cautious approach to circulatory stimulation at predicted metastasis sites might be appropriate, especially if they are located superficially - an example would be the axillary lymph nodes in breast cancer. This type of precaution has limited value, however, since most metastatic patterns involve the vital organs, and it is virtually impossible to limit the higher rate of blood flow these experience from an increase in the general circulation.

Summary of Metastasis Risk Information

In summary, it can be seen that the highest risk correlation probably occurs with firm direct contact or other strong stimuli applied on or near a tumour, with greatest concern arising if the tumour is close to the skin surface. This risk is greatly offset by the likelihood that should cells be released by such means, their odds of survival are still extremely slim.

The massage therapist's best course of action would be to obtain as much information as possible about the location of known tumours and avoid deep pressure and other intense local modalities. In the most conservative view, accessible predicted metastasis sites could also be approached with caution.

Fears about the risks from increased circulation of blood and lymph are probably unfounded. In fact, the effects of massage therapy may well mitigate against the survival of cancer cells moving in these media.

Because absolute statements cannot be made based on the information currently available, the massage therapist, the physician, and the client need to contemplate the risks in each case. The cancer type and progression, the client's degree of immune system function, medical treatments in progress, remission period or cancer-free time frame, possible massage treatment related risks, and the client's attitude and beliefs about the purpose of massage therapy in the treatment program should all be taken into consideration. As benefits are weighed against possible risks, the right to informed consent to treatment rests with the person with cancer.

How Does Massage Therapy Interact with Medical Treatment?

Surgery

In any case involving recent surgery, care must be taken not to disrupt the healing process. Gentle application of massage and hydrotherapy modalities can help reduce pain and inflammation and enhance circulatory efficiency as well as overall relaxation and comfort. The massage therapist must take steps to avoid promoting infection or any disruption of unsealed wounds. On-site manual techniques must be applied only after initial healing of the incision (normally 10-14 days) and with the understanding that healing of subcutaneous tissues will be ongoing for several weeks.

When the surgery has been undertaken as part of a cancer treatment protocol, there are additional considerations for the massage therapist. Surgery is a major shock to the body and places a strain on what may already be compromised immune function. When cancerous growths are removed, the surgeon cannot be absolutely certain of having excised all the malignant cells. This is the reason why a portion of the adjacent normal tissue is usually taken. The tissue disruption associated with surgery can have the effect of stimulating activity in any remaining malignant cells. The surgery and its related processes may also cause cancerous cells to be propelled into the general circulation. This volatility of the immediate post-surgery period makes it a vulnerable one for the client. Consultation with the surgeon or oncologist is essential in order to weigh the advantages and disadvantages of early massage intervention, and to ascertain the best time to begin treatment. A gentle relaxation focused treatment which avoids the surgical region may be appropriate soon after the surgery; more standard types of general and local treatment may not. It is important to have medical approval to proceed at this stage.

Tissue healing may not take place at the expected rate. The effects of the cancer and cancer therapies (which are often concurrent with post-surgical healing) include slowing of cellular repair processes, immunosuppression, malnutrition, and the possibility of clotting abnormalities. In addition to consulting with medical personnel as needed, the massage therapist must be alert for signs of possible deviation from what would be considered normal post-surgical healing. Such alertness would include close observation for decline in the skin condition, high or low temperature of the tissues, unexpected onset or increase of inflammation, increased or unresolved bruising or swelling, and pain which appears greater than expected or is otherwise worrisome. When such signs are present, medical consultation is necessary.

The likelihood of post-surgical infection is greater. With ill-considered therapy, the massage therapist may promote infection or cause spread of a pathogen that is already present. When an infection becomes established in tissues undergoing repair, tissue healing essentially stops until the infection is resolved. It is important to keep in mind, once the infection is over, that subcutaneous structures can be at a much earlier stage of healing than the time frame might otherwise indicate. Deeper pressures, or techniques which involve pulling on the surface, may traction underlying structures to a degree that they are not ready to tolerate, and should be introduced with caution.

Any indication of thrombosis should result in suspension of local massage therapy. Depending on the thrombus location, massage may be completely contraindicated until the problem has been medically treated. Similarly, if blood clotting is suppressed, massage may promote excessive bruising or disrupt tissue repair processes.

Cancer surgeries may involve extensive loss of functional tissue. It is important to ascertain what has been done and to have a reasonable idea of how the remaining tissue systems have been affected. For example, if a kidney has been removed, is the other kidney functioning well? Is it able to handle the effects of the massage techniques and/or hydrotherapy applications in the proposed treatment plan?

Some cancer surgeries are very extensive and deforming, requiring a tremendous emotional adaptation. This type of adjustment takes place in stages, and the massage therapist, who is seeing and perhaps touching the altered tissues, will need to be able to sustain an accepting and therapeutic presence. The client is trusting the massage therapist, as a health care professional, to help with the adjustment to his or her new body. It should also be remembered that intervening years do not always guarantee that an individual has accepted the deformity or the loss. Touch may elicit emotional responses, even years later.

Treatment of surgical scars, even older ones, should be considered in the light of risk of dislodging metastasizing cells. While the likelihood is not great, it is possible for malignant tissue to remain contained within an area of scarring. It is also possible for cancers to re-grow. Most cancers (breast cancer is a notable exception) are considered cured after five symptom-free years. A massage therapist treating someone during the years between diagnosis and cure will be uncertain about the status of the cancer. Wherever possible, an opinion should be sought from the oncologist or current family practitioner.

Radiation

Radiotherapy programs may extend over weeks and perhaps months, usually in 'on and off' intervals. Are there any guidelines for the massage therapist about how to interact compatibly with this type of treatment protocol? Unfortunately, to date no studies have been undertaken which would help clarify the ideal treatment relationship. We must proceed by exercising our best judgement given the known factors.

Radiation is focused as specifically as possible on identified tumour sites, and does not automatically preclude massage treatment of non-irradiated tissues. However, general symptoms like fatigue and nausea may delay massage therapy or alter the treatment approach.

Massage treatment of recently irradiated tissues poses some serious concerns; it must be considered very carefully and with full medical consultation. In the 'on' phases of a treatment program, the skin and other normal tissues are being damaged. Radiation injury has a progressive nature due to the slow release of free radicals in the affected tissues. (Consider the way a sunburn develops during the day or so following the exposure.) Depending on the body part or angle of irradiation, there may be a burn on the 'exit' surface as well.

The person receiving radiation therapy is prohibited from using most lubricants on the affected skin surface(s) because of the risk of increasing the burn damage. The massage therapist must take careful note of the instructions which have been given. One will encounter a range of medical approaches from prohibition of any substances except talcum powder, to permission to apply a special cream only, to limited use of water at skin temperature. Any scratching or rubbing (no matter how desired) is typically strongly discouraged.

It would seem reasonable to decide upon the following guidelines:

- seek medical consultation about the advisability of on-site work at any time during the treatment protocol
- comply with all restrictions on lubrication and touch
- pay careful attention to infection control
- completely avoid any on-site approaches during 'on' phases, with a two to three day wait into the 'off' phase to allow the burning process to subside
- consider carefully the healing needs of the skin and superficial tissues for at least the next 7-10 days, for example, avoid excessive 'tugging' on neighbour tissues
- no on-site work at any time when the skin surface is blistered or 'broken'
- wait 7-10 days following skin repair before beginning any focused specific on-site massage work
- have an ongoing awareness of tissue damage at the site, some of which will resolve and some become permanent

In the long term, previously irradiated skin may continue to be sensitive to sun, pressure, hot/cold, and other stimuli for many years. Joints frequently experience ongoing arthritic changes, and fascial structures (for example, tendons) may be permanently weakened. Bones, especially more fine bones like ribs, may be less resilient to pressure. Any history of radiation therapy should signal the massage therapist to carefully consider the current status of the affected tissues.

With respect to the potential for radiation injury to the therapist, it is generally believed that being with and touching someone who has received radiation therapy does not pose any significant risk. The exception would be an individual with an implanted radioactive source. This form of treatment is used rarely and always in a controlled hospital environment. Massaging under these circumstances would be risky for the massage therapist and would be prohibited by hospital policy.

Chemotherapy

With chemotherapy, unless regional methods are being used (in which case considerations analogous to those for radiation might be most appropriate), the massage therapist must be aware that the treatment effects are generalized. For example, the tendency of chemotherapy to damage rapidly reproducing tissues types means that skin and blood vessels are likely to be more fragile throughout the body.

Once again, the schedule of chemo treatments will typically be 'on' and 'off', with most individuals experiencing cycles of illness and recovery.

The massage therapist must consider the possibility that massage treatment could have a debilitating effect. This type of enervation response might result from:

- the potential for more rapid metabolization of the cytotoxic agent, making the person feel more ill
- overtaxing the fatigued individual when a rest period could be more beneficial
- overload on vital organ systems

Medical consultation is important to ensure that the timing and design of the massage treatment plan maximizes the safety and wellbeing of the client.

Some distinction is appropriate between relaxation enhancing touch (light massage) and a longer duration multiple component massage treatment. The latter is probably too taxing during and immediately following 'on' phases of chemotherapy. However, some nursing research has been conducted on the effects of "slow stroke back massage" during chemotherapy treatments to reduce nausea, anxiety, and muscle tension. Such studies[17,18,19] have examined the effects of gentle stroking back massage, averaging 3-10 minutes in duration, on the symptoms experienced. Consistently, subjects report reductions in nausea, anxiety, and overall symptom distress, along with an improved sense of wellbeing. In one study (Sims, 1986) this result appeared to be enhanced in clients with previous massage experience. Massage therapists could therefore offer this type of modified treatment to clients in chemotherapy, or show their family members how.

It may be fitting to incorporate a 2-3 day rest period before beginning more standard forms of massage therapy with someone just completing an 'on' phase of chemotherapy. A more extended period of rest or modified treatment may be advisable if the individual is particularly ill or debilitated. The appropriateness of treatment should be considered in a fresh light after each 'on' phase of a chemotherapy protocol, since the client may be more ill or weakened after, for example, the fifth session than the first. More vital organ system dysfunction may also be present.

As the person recovers after completion of a chemotherapy protocol it should be kept in mind that fatigue and low energy levels may persist for some time. As well, permanent joint degeneration may have occurred, and clinically significant vital organ damage may be present.

Other considerations are consistent with the general guidelines for massage treatment which follow shortly.

What is Good Case History Taking in a Cancer Case?

Case history taking involves asking specific and relevant questions and making observations. This process is most emphasized before the treatment plan is initiated, but must be continuous. Ongoing evaluation is particularly important in cancer cases because there are many changing factors which must be examined as the cancer and the treatment protocols follow their course. Questions are asked of the prospective client, medical personnel, and perhaps family members.

What follows is a group of information categories which should be included in the evaluation of a potential client who has cancer.

Case History Question Categories

1. **General Health History:** Any pertinent concurrent or past injuries or diseases; age and general health status; fitness level.

2. **Type and Stage of the Cancer:** Cancer type; history of progression; location of known tumour(s); regional lymph node involvement; client's and physician's opinion of prognosis/stage and metastasis status; usual metastasis pattern for the cancer; physician's opinion of risk of massage therapy promoting metastasis in any way (ask specific questions about components of the proposed treatment plan).

3. **Client's Goals for Massage Treatment:** Does the potential client have a realistic view of what massage can offer? Are there goals that you can mutually agree upon and share? Are they consistent with the massage therapy scope of practice?

4. **Medical Treatments - To Date and Projected:** Use the information provided in this booklet as a starting point to develop a set of specific questions about the treatment(s) used in the case. Research at the library and consult with other professionals as needed. Ask about time frames, how to interact with ongoing therapies, current side effects, or permanent complications. Take note of any restrictions mandated by physicians and ask specific questions related to the therapy you propose to do.

5. **Current Signs and Symptoms:** Put together the basics from this text and your research and ask as many specific questions as seem suited to the case. In

answer to a general question the person may forget a specific which is important to you. Make sure to ask about symptoms throughout the body, especially with disseminated cancer or recent chemotherapy. Ask at each meeting about new changes.

6. **The Person's Stress Levels, Support System:** Tactful questioning will most likely be experienced as concern and professional interest. Most people with cancer experience high levels of stress, and stress can have a negative impact on cancer recovery. Permit the client the choice not to answer questions if they are perceived as too personal. Observe for general mood and energy level, since your treatment approach may need to be altered in response to 'good' and 'bad' days.

7. **Medications:** In addition to direct treatment, medications may be prescribed for symptom relief. There are many possibilities of drugs the client could be taking which have an impact on massage treatment planning. These include: analgesics, tranquillizers or muscle relaxants, anti-inflammatories, sleeping pills, and so on. Keep current about medication changes.

8. **General Status of Body Symptoms:** Be as specific as possible in checking for indicators of vital organ failure - seek medical opinion as needed. Also, ask about nutrition levels, digestive symptoms, edema, blood pressure, strength and sensation changes.

9. **Pain Levels:** When pain is present, get a description of the pain: intensity, location, type; constant or intermittent; what makes it better or worse; effect of being touched; treatments to date; how pain medications affect mood, alertness, and ability to give feedback.

10. **Observation of Tissue Status:** Assess skin, scars, all structures in the vicinity of surgery and radiation treatments, joints (appearance and range of motion), edema.

11. **Current Activity and Exercise Levels, Common Hydro Practices:** Often you can take your guide from the types of daily stresses the person's body currently tolerates and gauge your proposed massage treatment accordingly. Ask about restrictions placed on these activities by the doctor.

12. **Special Consent:** Seek specific permission for treatment of scars, amputations, in the vicinity of ostomies, and so on. Requesting massage therapy does not confer blanket consent to expose or touch these parts unless the person wishes. Such consent should be renewed for each treatment.

What Does Massage Therapy Have to Offer?

The benefits massage therapy offers are significant ones. They could be summarized as follows:

- enhanced physical processes, for example more efficient circulation, improved skin condition

- symptom relief to prevent or reduce the need for additional medications (for example anti-emetic, anti-anxiety), and in cases where the medications could be contraindicated in combination with other therapies or poorly tolerated in the client's current state of health

- with some restrictions as previously given, relief of symptoms caused by surgery, radiation, and chemotherapy

- pain reduction/control

- improved mobility, lessening of secondary musculoskeletal effects

- improved quality of scarring, reduction of discomforts associated with scarring

- relaxation and reduction of stress and anxiety, with a variety of potential related benefits to healing and immune functions

- help with body acceptance

- time spent in a safe relationship with a good listener

More can be said about the last points. The medical literature contains expressions of increasing concern about the impact on patient health and cancer progression of the tremendous stress load associated with the cancer diagnosis and cancer treatment. In 1970, Dr. M. Bard, a contributor to a book entitled **Where Medicine Fails**, wrote: "The cancer patient is a person under a special and severe form of stress... all too many individuals are technically cured of their disease but left with an incapacitating psychological injury."[20] As more is learned about the relationship between stress and the resilience of body systems, more practitioners are becoming concerned about the effect high stress levels could have in hampering cancer recovery. Dr Carl Simonton writes extensively about this issue in his book **Getting Well Again**.[21]

Emphasis on the benefits of relaxation, focusing, and visualization of desired outcomes as an enhancement of treatment and recovery is now part of many mainstream cancer treatment protocols. Along with nutritional therapy and acupuncture, these adjunctive therapies are receiving more study and approval.

Massage functions very compatibly as part of this multidimensional type of treatment program. Massage therapy can introduce or strengthen the experience of relaxation and help the individual learn to achieve a relaxed state. Regular massage offers an interval of deep relaxation as a routine aspect of the person's schedule.

Clinical observation suggests that the regular experience of massage enhances the relaxation achieved in subsequent treatments and may lengthen the duration of the effect. Being massaged also serves as an excellent backdrop to enhance visualization or meditation for some clients.

Some people choose massage therapy as part of their treatment program because they find that they have come to feel alienated from their bodies as a result of the many distressing repercussions of cancer and cancer treatment. Massage can help create a bridge between the level of the physical body and the larger realm of personal integration and wellbeing.

A Nursing Study of Interest to Massage Therapists

A study reported in the nursing journal **Image** explored the efficacy of 'slow stroke back massage' in creating relaxation in hospice clients, most of whom were cancer patients. In her preliminary literature review the author makes reference to studies which have shown that seriously ill people are touched less frequently, and that a patient's diagnosis can reduce the amount he or she is touched by nurses. She also cites studies which demonstrate that massage induces relaxation and, in turn, that relaxation can reduce the need for pharmacologic pain control.

Given these background assumptions, a study was designed for a hospice setting to see if clear indicators could be observed demonstrating that massage could create a significant relaxation response in their clients.

There were 30 subjects, 16 males and 14 females, all older than 18, with prognoses of 6 months or less to live. None employed regular relaxation practices. The back massages were given by nurses according to a protocol frequently used in 'slow stroke back massage' studies. The subjects welcomed the treatments and showed "eagerness" to participate in the study.

All participants demonstrated statistically significant post-massage reductions in heart rate and systolic and diastolic blood pressures. These factors were still dropping 5 minutes after the massage, which was as long as measurement was done. Skin temperature increases were observed post-treatment; the skin temperature also continued to rise in the 5 minutes recorded after the massage.

The study results were considered very favourable and further exploration of the benefits of massage was recommended.

Meek SS, **Effects of Slow Stroke Back Massage on Relaxation in Hospice Clients**, IMAGE: Journal of Nursing Scholarship, Volume 25, Number 1, Spring 1993, pp. 17-21

Are There Special Concerns For Palliative Care?

Once the individual has widely disseminated cancer, or is considered to be in the terminal stages of the disease, many of the concerns associated with massage treatment planning diminish. As well, medical treatments become less interventionist and more focused on support and symptom relief, therefore more compatible with ongoing massage therapy.

Some principles are useful to keep in mind:

1. The primary goal of massage treatment in advanced cancers is comfort and enhancement of quality of life. The gentlest simplest techniques are often the most effective.

2. The body systems are weakening and close observation is necessary to ensure treatment adaptations are made as needed.

3. The person may be in severe pain. At this stage touch can sometimes increase the sensation of pain. The situation can vary from visit to visit and requires flexibility. Strong pain medication may significantly impair the client's ability to give reliable feedback about the treatment.

4. Regular contact with the medical team will help keep you current about medication and health status changes.

5. With reduced activity and cachexia, the person becomes increasingly susceptible to decubitus ulcers. The massage therapist can assist with prevention by working on maintaining good skin lubrication and good circulation to the skin, especially over bony areas on which the client routinely sits or lies. It should be noted that recent research indicates that massage of the affected skin is not advised once the early stage redness of a bedsore begins - in fact on-site massage can speed the skin breakdown at this point.[22]

6. The person may want to talk about death, or issues related to being ready for death. You may need to seek support if you are uncomfortable or feel unprepared to take part in this type of conversation.

7. As people approach death, their investments in ongoing relationships are usually slowly withdrawn. This is a normal part of letting go and should not be taken as a personal rejection.

Are There Some General Guidelines for Massage Therapy Treatment Adaptations?

1. **Give Serious Consideration to the Risk of Disrupting Tumours.** Discuss this issue and the proposed treatment plan with the oncologist. Do not proceed if the risk seems substantial. Be conservative in approach, avoiding direct pressure on known tumour sites. Be cautious with local hydrotherapy and mobilization techniques - avoid use if in doubt. Clarify tissue status following surgery and other medical treatments. Ensure that the client is as fully informed as possible about the effects of massage therapy before giving consent for treatment.

2. **Respond Honestly and with Integrity to the Person Involved.** Many of the beneficial effects of massage are premised on an open, trusting, safe client/therapist relationship; there is nothing to be gained by proceeding if the therapist is upset, pessimistic, or uncomfortable. The massage therapist must self monitor for reactions to cancer itself (especially if significant personal history is involved), to disfigurement, to prolonged illness, and to death. A well handled referral is better than attempting to mask undermining feelings and reactions. Supervision or psychotherapy may be important for the therapist who chooses to proceed.

3. **Do Not Feel Pressured Into Giving Treatment.** Massage treatment is not always appropriate. Going against your better judgement may weigh heavily given the serious health concerns involved. Take the time to get the information you need and to have conversations with the client about your mutual goals. You are the person in the situation who is expert on the application of massage therapy. Your judgement, while tempered by the client's wishes and medical information, is what you must rely on.

4. **Consider the Timing of Your Treatments in Relation to Medical Treatment Modalities.** Review the information in the earlier section **How Does Massage Therapy Interact With Medical Treatment?** Consult with the medical professionals involved, and carefully consider the client's level of fatigue, nausea, and general malaise with an eye to whether massage will be helpful and when it might have an enervating effect.

5. **Treat According to the Symptoms Present and the Condition of the Person and the Tissues.** No guidelines can adequately cover the possible range of occurrences in cancer. Be prepared to adapt as you go, and never hesitate to consult with the client, the family, the physician, or your research library. The client's emotional state may affect the type of massage treatment that is suitable on any given day.

6. **Be Aware of Tissue Fragility.** The cancer itself and the medical treatment modalities commonly used can cause tissue fragility, reduce repair capability, and predispose to hemorrhage and thrombosis. Any part of (including skin) the body may be affected. Skin quality and resilience are frequently compromised. Careful observation, good case history taking and consultation, and cautious introduction of massage, hydrotherapy, and exercise techniques are important. Keep in mind that the presence of infection adds to tissue repair time. As the cancer advances, cachexia can significantly increase tissue susceptibility to injury.

7. **Be Cautious About Infection and Fever.** The body fighting cancer is susceptible to hard-to-control episodes of fever and infection. Massage may promote the spread of infection. It may also overwhelm the body's resources if fever is present. Medical consultation is essential and the massage therapist should avoid treatment unless the situation is clearly under control.

8. **Consider Vital Organ System Failure.** Reduced systems function may have effects which are important for the massage therapist to consider. For example, liver, kidney, lung, and heart failure can all promote high blood pressure. Good case history taking and ongoing monitoring should include awareness of systemic changes. Remember that organ failure can be a chronic process. Keep track of what the client learns in regular medical check-ups. If you consider it appropriate to work toward vigorous full body treatment or large scale hydrotherapy applications, proceed toward such goals slowly and cautiously.

9. **Keep Track of the Client's Medications.** Massage impacts on the uptake of some drugs. Consultation with the doctor about treatment adaptations may be appropriate. In addition, some of the drugs prescribed (see **What Is Good Case History Taking?** on pages 30 and 31) affect the tissues in ways that require adjustments to your massage treatment approach.

10. **Be Aware of Sensory Losses or Impaired Awareness of Pain and Discomfort.** The impairment may be caused by cancer-related neurological damage, drug-induced mood, alertness, or sensory changes, sequelae of surgery or other treatment, or perhaps depression or near-death withdrawal. If you perceive that the client's feedback may be unreliable, proceed with extra caution.

11. **Monitor the Effects of Your Treatments.** Question the client carefully about the effects of each previous treatment and adapt to ensure the appropriateness of your ongoing treatment approach.

Cancer Case Studies

Case Study Questions

Case 1

You have a regular client, a 52 year old woman who has been seeing you for four years for relaxation work and treatment of neck and back pain related to a car accident which occurred five years ago. She has a deep left-side breast lump which was recently discovered as a result of a routine mammogram. She comes to see you in a highly distressed state two days after hearing this news and three days before her scheduled biopsy and possible mastectomy. She does not know whether she has cancer but has the impression that her situation does not look good to the doctors.

a) She really feels in need of receiving her massage. How do you proceed?

b) She tells you that you are someone she has come to trust and asks if you will continue treating her, assuming she does have cancer. How do you respond?

She does have breast cancer, and the surgeon proceeds directly to full mastectomy and regional lymph node sampling. The cancer was of a size and type which predicts metastasis may have already occurred, and lymph node involvement was confirmed. Radiation and chemotherapy are being planned, as well as bone scans and other diagnostic tests. Her first chemotherapy session is scheduled in three weeks time. The intubation (placement of a drainage tube endotracheally during general anaesthetic, with the neck extended and usually rotated to one side) has caused her upper back and neck pain to reappear, and her stress level is high. She asks you to arrange to treat her at home one week after the surgery.

a) What information do you need to have in order to make a decision about massage treatment at this time?

b) If you do decide to treat her how would you design the treatment? What aspects would you eliminate or modify?

c) If you decide not to treat her, how would you explain this decision to her?

Her projected chemotherapy program is one day per month for six months. However, the interval between the first and second sessions will be six weeks in order to incorporate radiation treatments. The doctor does not object to massage therapy during this time frame.

a) What type of massage treatment cycle would you consider appropriate?

She is given radiation once a week for five weeks during the interval between her first and second chemotherapies. You mutually agree to postpone massage therapy until after she finishes the radiation series because she is finding the process painful and exhausting. Her reaction to the treatment is very intense - her chest wall is burned and inflamed, with the surgical site showing recovery delay. The skin is blistered and oozing in several places. She is in a lot of pain and is very tired and depressed. Her second chemo session is postponed for two weeks to give her some recovery time.

a) How do you react, both as a person and as a health care practitioner, to her pain and distress?

b) Do you need more information at this point? How are your massage treatments affected?

Three months after completing the sixth chemotherapy session she is feeling much more resilient physically and her cancer status seems good. She confides that her husband, who has been "like a rock" during her illness, isn't responding well to her renewed interest in sexual intimacy and throughout has not been very comfortable looking at or touching her chest. She would rather not have more surgery and for the moment has decided against breast reconstruction. She thinks that intense massage work on the scar might improve its appearance as well as help reduce the edema in her arm (she has been wearing an elastic arm bandage) and improve the shoulder's range of motion. You have been doing more focused work on her neck and back lately, but have not addressed the mastectomy scar nor attempted to increase the mobility of her shoulder, which is limited by 90% in abduction, and by roughly 45% in external rotation and flexion/extension.

a)   What complications could develop because of her edema and limited mobility?

b)   What do you need to know, and how do you proceed in deciding about her new treatment requests?

c)   How do you respond to her comments about her husband?

Case 2

You are approached for treatment by a 28 year old man who three years ago had his right kidney removed and a short section of his jejunum re-sectioned because of cancer. Several lymph nodes were also excised. After the surgery he spent six months in a combined radiation and chemotherapy protocol. Currently, he appears to be in very good health with no evidence of cancer present. He sees his doctor every six months. His latest check-up was five weeks ago.

He has joined a health club and is working at getting more fit. He would like your help with the extensive scar tissue - he finds it restrictive and uncomfortable during most types of exercise. On examination, you find that the scar extends from front to back on the entirety of his right side, arcing along his lower ribs. The scar is strongly adhered to deeper tissues in several locations.

a) What information do you want to have in your decision-making and treatment planning process?

b) In your opinion are there any contraindications or special considerations in this case?

Case 3

You are approached by a friend to treat his father, who is a 78 year old man with advanced prostatic cancer. He has extensive spinal, colon, and liver metastasis, and has been told that he has 4-6 weeks to live. The cancer was diagnosed four years ago. Given that it had already spread within the abdomen, no surgery was done. His cardiovascular health was assessed as too poor to proceed with chemotherapy.

In the interim he has had one surgery to remove a bowel obstruction. This was done four months ago. His back pain is quite severe, necessitating regular morphine. He is also on blood pressure medication, the dosage having been increased twice since the liver metastasis became apparent two months ago. His degree of consciousness and alertness varies from very good to quite poor, and his disposition ranges from quite sociable to withdrawn and irritable and impatient. He has a strongly expressed wish to die at home.

Although a tall man he weighs 110 pounds at this point. He has considerable ascites and lower limb edema. He does not have a colostomy.

a) What information do you want to have to make sure that you are sufficiently informed about this case?

Assuming you decide to work with this client,

a) How would you address the consent issues involved?

b) What do you see as your role in the team of family members and health care workers treating him in his home?

c) Are there specific considerations about working with his cachexia? What treatment adaptations do you consider necessary?

d) Do you as a therapist feel emotionally ready to address this case? What are the issues for you?

e) Give an outline of the treatment plan you would consider suitable to try with him in your first few sessions.

Case Study Discussion

Case 1

a)   She really feels in need of receiving her massage. How do you proceed?

Avoid deep or focused work in the vicinity of her axillary, pectoral, and subclavicular lymph nodes to offset any risk of mobilizing metastasic cells. If you have been doing breast massage, avoid this treatment. These precautions may be over-cautious, but now that you know she may have breast cancer the situation is not the same as it was last week, and it is better to wait for clear information.

Avoid acting as though you believe she does or does not have cancer. Take a wait-and-see approach, in a warm and supportive manner. Inform her that the treatment design changes are probably too cautious, but in your opinion a good idea until you both know what is going on.

It is too alarming, as well as unnecessary, to avoid treating her altogether. Given the stress she is under, design a non-specific relaxation treatment which concentrates on reducing her stress and allows her to talk or not to talk as she wishes.

b)   She tells you that you are someone she has come to trust and asks if you will continue treating her, assuming she does have cancer. How do you respond?

You have to look at what she is asking of you. At this stage she wants to know if you will stand by her, and if she can count on some things going on as before. For some practitioners this is an easy commitment to make right away. If that is the case for you, go ahead and say yes, with the proviso that you would always want to be working within medical guidelines.

For others there may be a sense of fear, or inadequacy. Perhaps you have a personal history related to breast cancer which makes you uncertain about your ability to stay completely professional. At this point, when it is not clear that she has breast cancer, voicing these reservations may seem like a cruel rejection, may be completely unnecessary, and would likely cause damage to your relationship no matter how they were stated. If you are uncertain, you need time to think and perhaps to seek advice. You may need more education, or you may need to establish an ongoing supervision relationship to support you while you address the issues her case brings to the surface in you. The best way to handle the situation at this point is to say that it is too soon to know how the doctors would decide to proceed if she does have cancer, and how massage would fit in to the overall treatment plan. Commit yourself to follow up with her after the biopsy, and to consult with her and her doctor(s) after the diagnosis is clear. Get permission to interact with her physician(s) and specifics about how to do so. In other words, commit yourself for the next stage. In the interim, do your best to clarify how to proceed for your own needs, and how best to discuss any negative decision with her should she be diagnosed with cancer.

a) What information do you need to have in order to make a decision about massage treatment at this time?

From the oncologist/surgeon (be prepared to follow up at the library), get as many specifics as you can about the type of cancer, its likely progression, possible metastasis sites, perceived success of the surgery, and upcoming treatment plans. Keeping in mind that the fact that the immediate post-surgical period is a vulnerable one for increased activity of any remaining cancer cells, get his or her opinion about whether massage and/or hydrotherapy might add to the risks at this time. In other words, are there reasons to avoid general or local treatment?

If you plan to proceed, ask about specifics in your proposed treatment plan. For example: Would it be appropriate to use warm/cool contrast hydrotherapy on her left arm? Should I avoid mobilizing her left shoulder at this stage? Doctors cannot be expected to be experts on the components of massage therapy treatments and will provide more useful information in response to specific questions.

Ask the client and her doctor about her current general health status, how she is recovering, her level of pain, the presence of any signs of infection, and medications she is taking. In particular, inquire about meds that could affect alter your treatment approach, for example analgesics, anti-inflammatories, anticoagulants, sleeping pills, and tranquillizers.

b) If you do decide to treat her how would you design the treatment? What aspects would you eliminate or modify?

Consider the following concerns:

* *It is too soon to do anything that would directly stress the surgical site (on-site massage, rigorous stretching or tractioning).*
* *There is a risk of promoting infection.*
* *There is a need for caution with respect to strong stimulation of blood flow through the surgical site (may be a thrombus present, blood vessels may not be sufficiently repaired, may promote cancer cell activity at this vulnerable point).*
* *A massage treatment that is too long or too stimulating may be overtaxing in her present state.*
* *Medications may be altering her perception of pain or her reflex responses.*

The treatment design should focus on relaxation and providing a sense of safety and wellbeing. It is not necessary that the treatment be a full body massage or an hour in length. Your work should be light and general in nature - avoid painful work and intense hydrotherapy and range of motion modalities. Check carefully for signs that she is uncomfortable, or is tiring or feeling overstressed by your work. Make sure she understands that she can modify or end the treatment if she becomes fatigued or feels that she has had enough work. Take into account the types of medication she is using and how they may be impacting on her feedback.

Be particularly careful about hygiene, especially in the vicinity of the surgical site.

Ask in what position she is most comfortable lying. Prone position will likely not be workable. Make sure sidelying on either side is comfortable before proceeding - she may need a pillow or towel between her left arm and her torso when lying on her right side. Elevate her left arm when she is supine.

The most cautious approach would be to give a soothing back massage if she can be positioned comfortably in sidelying, followed by light neck work in supine and a reflex type of treatment of the hands and feet. This may be enough for the first treatment. Do not proceed with in-depth neck work unless she seems particularly fit and you have medical permission. I would probably be inclined to wait, even with her request and the doctor's okay, to see how she responds to this first treatment before getting into the deeper neck work.

c)   If you decide not to treat her, how would you explain this decision to her?

At this stage I would express the opinion that it is too soon, that the massage may be too taxing, or that you would prefer to take a conservative approach toward her safety and wait a while longer. Address the issue in a manner which she would receive as both honest and supportive, based on your previous relationship. If the doctor has refused permission for massage, make sure that you do not come across as antagonistic toward the doctor. She needs to feel that her team is working together in her best interest.

a)   What type of massage treatment cycle would you consider appropriate?

First of all, if you have come to the conclusion that you will be personally unable to treat her, you must communicate this to her as soon as she is reasonably back to normal following the surgery but before she begins chemotherapy. You must honestly present your concerns, making sure that she understands that the issue is yours, and not related to any problem or shortcoming of hers. To complete the process you must provide her with at least one (preferably several) appropriate referral to another massage therapist.

If you are proceeding, what will likely make most sense is to begin by offering to come once to her home or the hospital to show family members/friends how to do the slow stroke type of soothing back massage that has been found to help with symptom relief during chemotherapy.

Establish a system of waiting 2 - 3 days following an 'on' phase before resuming treatment. Make sure that she knows that she can delay more days on short notice if she doesn't feel ready.

Be aware that after each round of chemo she may take longer to bounce back. Re-check after each round for tissue fragility, joint degeneration, and vital organ system status.

Be aware of her depressed immune status - hygiene concerns are paramount. As well, you must avoid exposing her to routine 'bugs' that you or your other clients may have.

Build slowly toward full length, more comprehensive types of treatment designs. Monitor her reactions from each previous treatment and incorporate more intense techniques and modalities gradually.

This is a time when many cancer patients benefit tremendously from joining a support group or finding another means of meeting regularly with others on the same journey. You may be able to make a good recommendation, or offer your support if she is hesitant to follow up on a suggestion from another member of her health care team. Your role will also have an important dimension of listening and offering the types of support which fall within your scope.

a) How do you react, both as a person and as a health care practitioner, to her pain and distress?

First, make sure that she is absolutely clear about her right to have or not have treatments, or to modify the length and focus of each treatment to suit how she feels and what she needs that day. She will need a sense of control, as well as a clear indication that you can adapt to changing needs and energy levels as she experiences them without her having to worry about letting you down.

Since you will not have seen her for a while, it is important to prepare yourself for the sight and smell of her tissue, as well as her depression and overall 'low' state. Ask friends who are nurses or who have otherwise had experience of someone at this stage of cancer treatment to describe to you what you are likely to encounter. Failing that, ask her doctor. Work in supervision or in other ways within your personal support system to make sure you feel ready to approach working with her in a calm and encouraging manner.

Your touch, and your warmth and energy are important resources for her, perhaps much more so than your technical skill. Keep this in perspective for yourself.

b) Do you need more information at this point? How are your massage treatments affected?

Make sure that you are clear about how to avoid causing or increasing infection – this is a major concern since she has open skin lesions and her immune system responses will be low.

This type of radiation exposure may directly damage the heart and left lung. Ascertain the current status of these organ systems before proceeding.

Check for new medications, or altered dosages.

Do not proceed with on-site and local work unless you have medical permission and until the skin has healed. Proceed cautiously since the skin and subcutaneous tissues will continue to be fragile for some time. Be aware that the upcoming chemo round will also affect her tissue repair.

Her emotional state and energy level are key factors in determining your treatment design at this time. She will probably be having 'good days' and 'bad days,' so her physical and emotional needs will vary greatly.

If you find yourself struggling to cope, make sure that you are receiving sufficient support. Ask yourself if you are taking on too much – is there a member of her health care team who provides counselling? Does she need a referral? Is she making use of the personal supports available to her? Are you in enough contact with the team to get any information or assistance you need?

a)   What complications could develop because of her edema and limited mobility?

* thoracic outlet syndrome
* carpal tunnel syndrome
* frozen shoulder
* sub-deltoid/sub-acromial bursitis
* painful trigger point syndromes
* arthritic changes in her neck, shoulder, elbow, wrist, and hand
* skin and soft tissue dystrophy, especially distally in the limb
* scoliosis, joint and muscle pain syndromes in her back and neck due to asymmetric usage

b)   What do you need to know, and how do you proceed in deciding about her new treatment requests?

You need a good assessment of her tissue status in the context of the type of work being considered. Is the surgical site skin and subcutaneous tissue well healed and stable enough for friction therapy? Can the tissues tolerate intense hot or cold applications? Are the underlying ribs weakened and therefore less resilient to pressure? What is her sensation like in the scarred tissue, and the arm and hand? Despite the edema, does she seem to have reasonably good proximal circulation? Has she been stretching her neck and left shoulder? How painful is it? How much day-to-day usage of her arm is comfortable?

Make sure you are up to date about her vital organ system status.

Check again on her medications. Anti-inflammatories, muscle relaxants and anticoagulants can all alter the tissue resilience to intense direct local treatment. It is possible that she is still taking analgesics, which may affect her ability to accurately experience tissue stress during rigorous treatment.

While the doctor's opinion should be sought, no one can really predict the metastasis risk at this stage, either in general, or as a result of the type of local massage work being considered. The risk is likely very low, but there are no guarantees. Discuss this with her in a balanced, completely open way. Individuals at this stage of cancer recovery are usually working within their own framework of choice, thinking carefully about safety factors in relationship to their need for a satisfying life and a renewed sense of control. It is essential to make sure that she is giving fully informed consent to treatment.

If all of the above factors look workable, try applying deep heat (wax may be best) followed by focused petrissage and frictions to a small area on an outer edge of the scar. The treatment area should be about a square inch. Check carefully for pain and tissue response. Follow this treatment with several moderate stretches which will apply normal stress to the treated area within her tolerance of shoulder range of motion. Then apply ice. Give her similar stretching to do at home. Ask her to take note of how the tissue looks and feels for the next few days. Assess at your next session. While some tenderness, inflammation, and local swelling might be expected, an acute flare-up, or a strong pain reaction, or achiness or swelling lasting beyond a couple of days would suggest waiting longer to start this type of treatment approach.

c) How do you respond to her comments about her husband?

Empathic listening is the limit of the massage therapist's scope in this situation. Resumption of their sexual relationship is often difficult after a long interval in which one partner in a couple has been ill. If you feel that you can make a good referral, and it seems appropriate to offer one, you could suggest marriage counselling. At all costs avoid expressing judgements of her husband's feelings or behaviour. Most relationships under this kind of stress will encounter rough spots - if you feel you can offer encouragement from your own knowledge or experience, do so in a general, supportive way. Do not make comments that could be construed as authoritative or offering professional advice.

Case 2

a) What information do you want to have in your decision-making and treatment planning process?

Since you know that his general health is good and there is no evidence of cancer, focus on determining the resilience of the tissues and structures that could be stressed by massage:

* How well is his remaining kidney functioning - are there any indicators that it is struggling with the increased workload? Is there any sign of damage from the cancer treatments? What is the doctor's opinion of his kidney resilience? Would intense hydrotherapy and massage treatment be too taxing?

* Is there any reduction in heart function? Are his heart and kidney able to maintain normal blood pressure? If his blood pressure is high, get specifics and ask about medication. Is there any edema or extremity tissue dystrophy? Is there any shortness of breath? Ask the case history questions which will assess for congestive heart failure.

* Check carefully that the ribs can withstand pressure in the locations where you would be working intensely on the scar. Similarly, check for radiation-related damage in the soft tissues, i.e., loss of or unreliable sensation, permanent weakness of the skin and/or underlying soft tissue structures.

Get specifics about the surgery: method of entry, how easily the healing progressed, if there were any problems with infection, the current status of the involved tissues.

Does he have an ileostomy? If yes, discuss how to maintain good hygiene, and how best to position him for treatment.

Medications?

What is his current fitness level? What are his activities of daily living (work, exercise, home hydro practices)? What are his fitness goals?

Assess him specifically for posture, range of motion, and pain on movement.

b) In your opinion are there any contraindications or special considerations in this case?

It is still important to ascertain his doctor's opinion of risk of metastasis, especially from direct work involving the surgical area. The client must be allowed to consider the risks, which although quite small, cannot be glossed over. You must discuss this issue in an open and balanced way and ensure that informed consent is obtained.

He may have cardiovascular and renal weaknesses that necessitate treatment adaptation. Largely, these adaptations would involve (depending on the degree of deficiency) reducing the size and temperature of hydrotherapy applications, avoiding large drainage strokes, working specific body areas in preference over full body treatment, exercising caution with the amount of pain caused during the treatment, and having an overall emphasis on relaxation and reduction of sympathetic activation.

There may be a need to adapt to poor tissue health and irregular sensation in the vicinity of the scar.

Case 3

a) What information do you want to have to make sure that you are sufficiently informed about this case?

You need a good evaluation of his vital organ system status, especially his cardiovascular system. Ask questions to elicit information about how his heart is functioning (his degree of congestive heart failure, in this case). Get specifics about his blood pressure - how high is it? Is this level steady or does it fluctuate? How well is the medication controlling it? How well does his heart adapt to pressure increases, given the possibility of massage increasing his blood pressure? What is his overall energy level and tolerance of exertion? Are mild types of hydrotherapy, for example, cool/warm compresses, okay to use?

Also, how are his kidneys? Given the medications and the high blood pressure, check on indicators of reduced kidney function.

Lung clearance is often suppressed by morphine. As well, it can be assumed that he has some degree of congestive heart failure, and therefore pulmonary edema. Check on the status of his breathing and lung function. Does he have dyspnea (impaired breathing) lying fully supine, or in any other position?

Given that massage treatment will be a stressor, the degree of function and level of resilience of his vital organ systems will determine whether you should massage at all, or how much modification is needed.

Get specifics about the surgery - what was done? How well have the tissues healed? In this case healing may be quite poor, and although it is unlikely that you will massage his abdomen in any rigorous way (because of the blood pressure), there may be an impact on his comfort levels in different positions.

You need to know about the medications he is taking - make sure you have a complete list. Research the effects of any with which you are not familiar. What are the combined side effects? To what extent do they affect his ability to give accurate feedback? With respect to his meds, are there better or worse times of the day to massage?

Is his pain level constant? Does he have good and bad times of day? When he is in a great deal of pain, does being touched lessen the pain or make it worse? Is he more comfortable in certain positions? Is there anything else that helps?

a) How would you address the consent issues involved?

As much as possible it is important to get a sense of the father's interest in and consent to massage treatment. Is it the son's idea? Does the father want massage? Try to find a time to visit, or to speak with the father on the telephone when he is alert. Do not have an expectation of giving a treatment if you see him in person. If he is expressing interest, speak gently about the fact that sometimes he is not as aware as at present. Would he mind being massaged at those times? What about when he is in a lot of pain? If you can get a reliable feel for his point of view, proceed accordingly. It would be inappropriate to proceed if he is mentally competent and refuses consent.

If it is clear that he cannot interact with you in a way that you feel confident constitutes informed consent to treatment, family consent is sufficient to proceed. Usually one individual has been given authority by the client to make this type of decision. I would suggest making an agreement with this person to give 2-3 conservatively designed treatments to see how the client responds and if he appears to be enjoying or not enjoying the work. It is also important to check carefully on his physical status during and after massage to see how beneficial the treatments are. If the signs are favourable, proceed with family consent to a more extended treatment plan.

At this stage of the case, the concern is finding a treatment level suited to his overall health status. Given the rate of advancement of his cancer, there is no significant concern about massage therapy promoting metastasis.

b) What do you see as your role in the team of family members and health care workers treating him in his home?

All members of this type of team are expected to be supportive of each other and work cooperatively together. A key aspect of this cooperation is prompt and clear communication of any health status or emotional state changes in the client. Although massage therapists are often more accustomed to working alone, it is important to function as part of the team, and therefore to see yourself as part of the support and information network the family and health care workers have formed for the care of the client. Another element of teamwork is exchange of ideas and treatment approaches based on the specific areas of expertise represented on the team.

In addition to providing massage yourself, you can show medical team and family members how to do simple massage treatments, based on what the client seems to enjoy. Gentle back massage, or hand and foot treatments, for example, might be more beneficial if received daily. As well, this type of contact often helps the family, and the nurses, to feel that they can offer warm and supportive care.

It may be appropriate, based on your agreement with the family, to provide massage for the team as well.

c) Are there specific considerations about working with his cachexia? What treatment adaptations do you consider necessary?

Given this client's extensive loss of tissue, it is important to establish how much pressure and stretch his muscles and connective tissues can tolerate. Proceed slowly and carefully.

The poor quality of the muscles and other tissues stabilizing his joints may lead to hypermobility and/or easy subluxation. Be cautious with position changes, with use of passive exercise modalities, and when positioning his body parts during the treatment.

The cachexic client is susceptible to bedsores (decubitus ulcers). Massage can be effective in helping to prevent them, so in a case like this it is important to focus on enhancing circulation and skin quality, especially over bony areas and in tissues on which he frequently lies or sits. However, once the early redness or skin deterioration of an ulcer has developed, careful avoidance of on-site massage or any modalities which will pull on the tissue and strict attention to hygiene are indicated.

d) Do you as a therapist feel emotionally ready to address this case? What are the issues for you?

Before taking this type of case it is important to check with yourself to see if you believe you can proceed in a calm and supportive professional manner. Do you need personal supervision or support? Have you considered how the client's state of health and imminent death will affect you? Do you have personal issues which might get in the way of your quality of care? If you do, does it make most sense to refer to someone else, or would it be best to move forward with good support?

In this case, where the potential client is a friend's father, it is also important to consider your relationship to the situation. Do you know the father well? If you do, does your existing relationship foster the kind of professional role you are considering undertaking? Would it be awkward in some way? What expectations does the son have of you and of massage? Are they realistic? How do you feel about committing to being a member of the palliative care team for this family?

e) Give an outline of the treatment plan you would consider suitable to try with him in your first few sessions.

In designing your first and subsequent treatments consider the following:

* Determine your treatment priorities based on how best to improve his comfort and quality of life.
* Does his physical status indicate strong caution about overstressing his heart? If yes, keep the treatment short (20-30 minutes) and use only soothing, reflex types of work. Incorporate more focused

massage to skin overlying bony prominencies, but keep it slow and rhythmical.

Given the blood pressure problem, maintain a relaxation focus at all times, and begin by treating the limbs. Work gradually to full body treatment, if at all. Even if his heart is moderately resilient, treatments should not exceed 40 minutes. Avoid any abdominal and neck work that would compress major blood vessels. Do not work simultaneously on both sides of his neck. Avoid large drainage strokes, as well as painful or stressful types of work.

Adapt your plan around positioning that is comfortable for him.

Hydrotherapy, if used at all, must be introduced gradually, with small applications of moderated temperatures.

His pain levels may fluctuate, and at times he may be more or less sensitive to being touched. His body will likely react differently from treatment to treatment. Some body parts may always be good to treat, while others may have to be considered optional depending on his reaction.

Be aware that, regardless of his ability to communicate verbally with you, your touch and your voice are sending him strong messages. Assume that on some level he is always aware of the quality of your interaction and your attentiveness to him and the treatment, as well as to conversations and atmosphere in the room. Keep the treatment environment as quiet, peaceful, and focused meaningfully on him as possible.

Always keep in mind the unreliability of his feedback, and his changing health status. Watch carefully for physical signs that he is being fatigued or overtaxed by the day's treatment. Be ready to stop massaging or change your plan.

REFERENCES

1. Woolf N: <u>Cell, Tissue and Disease</u>, 2nd ed., London, Bailliere Tindall, p. 361

2. Bonica J: *Cancer Pain*, Klatersky J & Staquet M, eds: <u>Medical Complications in Cancer Patients</u>, pp. 87-88

3. Hildebrand J: *Neurological Disorders in Cancer Patients and Their Treatment*, <u>Klatersky J & Staquet M, eds: Medical Complications in Cancer Patients</u>, p.51

4. Sherman C: *Principles of Surgical Oncology*, Kahn S, Love R, Sherman C, & Chakravorty R, eds: <u>Concepts in Cancer Medicine</u>, p. 304

5. Wolberg W: *Metastasis*, Kahn S, Love R, Sherman C, & Chakravorty R, eds: <u>Concepts in Cancer Medicine</u>, p.149

6. Information abstracted from Kaiser H: *Comparative Importance of the Lymphatic System During Neoplastic Progression: Lymphohematogenous Spreading*, Goldfarb R, ed: <u>Fundamental Aspects of Cancer</u>, Cancer Growth and Progression Series, Volume 1

7. Information abstracted from Netland P & Zetter B: *Tumor Cell Interactions with Blood Vessels During Cancer Metastasis*, Goldfarb R, ed: <u>Fundamental Aspects of Cancer</u>, Cancer Growth and Progression Series, Volume 1

8. Fidler IJ: *Metastasis: Quantatative Analysis of the Distribution and Fate of Tumor Emboli Labeled with 125I-5-iodo-2'-deoxyuridine*. This study and five others supporting the same finding are reviewed in Netland P & Zetter B: *Tumor Cell Interactions with Blood Vessels During Cancer Metastasis*, Goldfarb R, ed: <u>Fundamental Aspects of Cancer</u>, Cancer Growth and Progression Series, Volume 1, p. 87

9. A review of numerous studies related to this subject can be found in

Netland P & Zetter B: *Tumor Cell Interactions with Blood Vessels During Cancer Metastasis*, Goldfarb R, ed: Fundamental Aspects of Cancer, Cancer Growth and Progression Series, Volume 1, pp. 84-97

10. Plesnicar S: *Mechanisms of Development of Metastases*, Critical Review in Oncogenesis, 1/2:176

11. Abramson D: *Questions and Answers*, Journal of the American Medical Association, 237/8:812

12. Simonton OC, Matthews-Simonton S & Creighton J: Getting Well Again, p. 222

13. Tope DM, Hahn DM, Pinkson B, *Massage Therapy: An Old Intervention Comes of Age*, 1994, Internet Source: ONCOLINK

14. Extensive review of related studies found in Netland P & Zetter B: *Tumor Cell Interactions with Blood Vessels During Cancer Metastasis*, Goldfarb R, ed: Fundamental Aspects of Cancer, Cancer Growth and Progression Series, Volume 1, p. 87

15. Extensive review of related studies in Varani J, McCoy JP & Ward PA: *The Attraction of Wandering Metastatic Cells*, Goldfarb R, ed: Fundamental Aspects of Cancer, Cancer Growth and Progression Series, Volume 1, pp. 73-83

16. *The Biology of Cancer*, notes from Spring, 1995 Biology of Cancer class at Berkeley, Internet Source: ONCOLINK

17. Scott D, Donahue D, Mastrovito R & Hakes D: *The Anti-Emetic Effect of Clinical Relaxation: Report of an Exploratory Pilot Study*, Journal of Psychosocial Oncology, Spring, 1983

18. Sims S: *Slow Stroke Back Massage for Cancer Patients*, NursingTimes, November, 1986

19. Warren K: *Will I be Sick, Nurse?*, Nursing Times, 84/12, 1988

20. Quoted by Krant M: *Psychological Aspects of Cancer Diagnosis*, Klastersky J & Staguet M, eds: Medical Complications in Cancer Patients, p.69

21. Simonton OC, Matthews-Simonton S & Creighton J: Getting Well Again,

22. US Department of Health and Human Services, *Pressure Ulcers in Adults: Prediction and Prevention*, Clinical Practice Guideline, Number 3, AHCPR Publication No. 92-0047, May 1992, p.3, p.19

BIBLIOGRAPHY

1. Abramson, D.I., "Questions and Answers." *JAMA*, Volume 237, Number 8, February 21, 1977

2. Bammer, K. and Newberry, B.H., *Stress and Cancer*. Toronto: C.J. Hogrefe Inc., 1981

3. Cooper, J.S. and Pizzarello, D.J., *Concepts in Cancer Care*. Philadelphia: Lea and Febiger, 1980

4. Ferrell-Torry, A.T. & Glick, O.J., "The Use of Therapeutic Massage as a Nursing Intervention to Modify Anxiety and the Perception of Cancer Pain." *Cancer Nursing*, Volume 16, Number 2, 1993

5. Goldfarb, R.H. ed., *Fundamental Aspects of Cancer*. Cancer Growth and Progression Series, Volume 1. Netherlands: Kluwer Academic Publishers, 1989

6. Higby, D.J., *Supportive Care in Cancer Therapy*. Boston: Martinus Nijhoff Publishers, 1983

7. Kahn, S.B. et al, *Concepts in Cancer Medicine*. New York: Grune & Stratton, 1983

8. Klastersky, J. and Staguet, M.J., *Medical Complications in Cancer Patients*. New York: Raven Press, 1981

9. Leighton, J., *The Spread of Cancer*. New York: Academic Press, 1967

10. Lokich, J.J. and Byfield, J.E., *Combined Modality Cancer Therapy*. Chicago: Precept Press, 1991

11. Meares, A., "Massage as an Adjunct to Meditation in the Psychological Treatment of Cancer." *Australia Physiotherapy*, Volume 26, Issue 1, February 1980

12. Meeks, S.S., "Effects of Slow Stroke Back Massage in Hospice Clients." *IMAGE: Journal of Nursing Scholarship*, Volume 25, Number 1, Spring 1993

13. Morra, M. and Potts, E., *Choices: Realistic Alternatives in Cancer Therapy*. New York: Avon, 1987

14. Plesnicar, S., "Mechanisms of Development of Metastases." *Critical Review in Oncogenesis*, Volume 1, Issue 2, 1989

15. Porth, C.M., *Pathophysiology*, 3rd ed. Philadelphia: J.B. Lippincott, 1990

16. Scott, D.W. et al., "The Anti-Emetic Effect of Clinical Relaxation: Report of an Exploratory Pilot Study." *Journal of Psychosocial Oncology*, Spring 1983

17. Simonton, O.C. et al, *Getting Well Again*. New York: Bantam, 1980

18. Sims, S., "Slow Stroke Back Massage for Cancer Patients." *Nursing Times*, November 19, 1986

19. Warren, K., "Will I Be Sick, Nurse?" *Nursing Times*, Volume 84, Number 12, March 23, 1988

20. Weinrich, S.P. & Weinrich, M.C., "The Effect of Massage on Pain in Cancer Patients." *Applied Nursing Research*, Volume 3, Number 4, 1990

21. Willis, R.A., *The Spread of Tumours in the Human Body*. London: Butterworths, 1973

22. Woolf, Neville, *Cell, Tissue and Disease*, 2nd ed. London: Baillière Tindall, 1988

INDEX

joint degeneration, 28, 29

lymph circulation, 22–3, 24
lymph drainage, 23
lymphogenous metastasis, 4, 19–20,
    22–3

malignant (definition), 4
malignant neoplasms, 8, 9
massage instruction (for family,
medical team), 29, 59
massage therapy
    as adjunctive therapy, 32–3
    benefits for cancer patients, 32–3
    cancer treatment adaptations,
    36–7
    principles for palliative care, 35
medications, 15, 31, 37, 50, 54
metastasis, 4, 7, 19–24
    cause of death, 19–20
    formation patterns, 24
    post-surgical, 25, 48, 49
    risk correlation with massage,
    21–4, 47, 54, 56
    from scar sites, 27
    stages, 21–4

neoplasia, 4, 8
neoplasm(s), 4, 7
nervous system complications, 11

oncologist, 4

pain
    as cancer symptom, 11
    case history questions about, 31
    control and reduction, 32, 34
    impaired awareness of, 37
palliative care, 4, 34, 35, 57–61
palliative surgery, 14
parenchyma, 4, 7
progenitor cells, 7

radiation sites, 15

radiation therapy, 4, 14–16, 27–8
relaxation treatments, 29, 33, 34, 47

scars, surgical, 26–7, 32
    treatment, 54, 56
skin
    breakdown, 35, 59–60
    care during radiation therapy, 27
    radiation site marks, 15
skin lesions, 11
slow stroke back massage, 29, 34, 51
stem cells, 7
stroma, 4, 7
support groups, 51
surgery, 14, 25–7
symptoms
    of cancer, 9–11
    case history questions, 30–1
    relief of, 22

therapists
    awareness of ominous signs, 25
    decision to treat cancer patients,
    48, 50–1, 60
    as member of palliative care
team, 59, 60
    personal support systems, 51, 52
    supervision or self-monitoring,
    36, 60
thrombosis, 26, 37
tissue
    assessment of, 53
    fragility, 37
    loss through surgery, 26
treatment designs
    palliative care, 60–1
    post-surgical, 49–51, 54
treatments, timing of, 27, 28, 29, 36
tumour(s), 4, 8
    cell shedding from, 20, 21–2
    risk of disrupting, 21–4, 36
    secondary site, 23–4
    signs and symptoms, 9
    surgical removal, 14